This Book Belongs to:

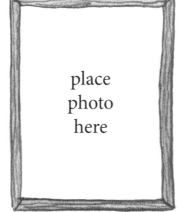

place
photo
here

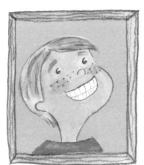

JAMIE

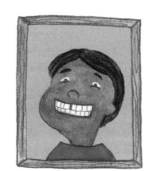

RAJ

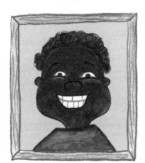

ELIJAH

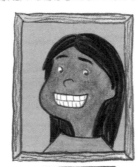

SELINA

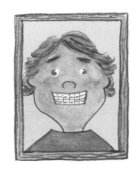

MASON

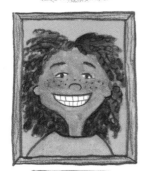

RUBY

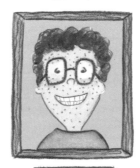

SAM

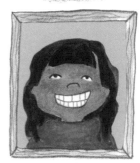

CAMILLA

For Finn.

This book is produced with papers certified by both FSC® and the
Rainforest Alliance™

Published by Chatwin Books

For orders & inquiries:
www.TheToothFairyExperience.com

Delta Dental of Washington
Seattle, Washington
www.DeltaDentalWa.com

ISBN: 978-1-63398-142-3

The CLEAN TEETH CLUB

a tooth fairy tale

BY KELLY RAE BAHR

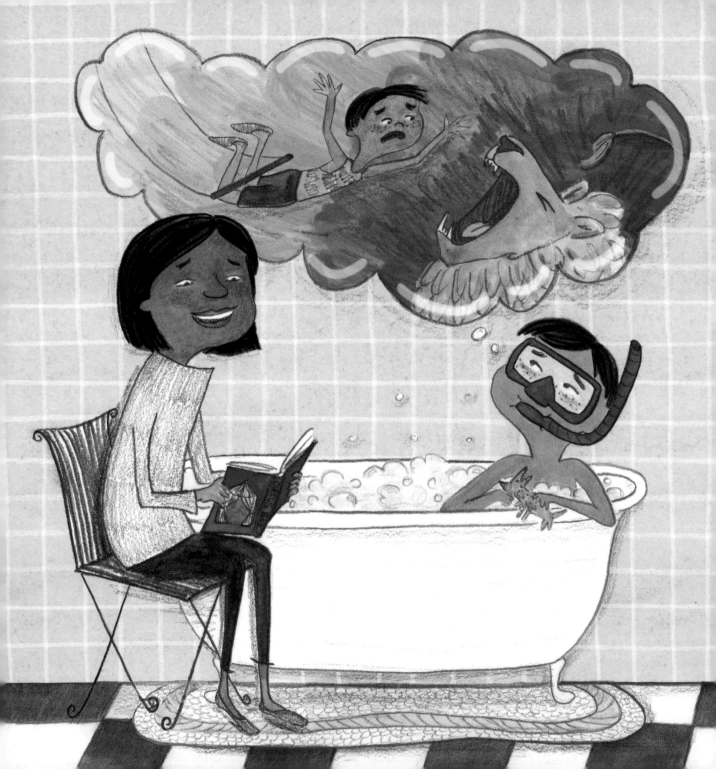

A boy named Tyler sat in the tub
and dreamed of joining a special club.
A cool kind of club, like a hiking group,
or a diving team, or a circus troupe.
No, thought Tyler, those aren't for me.
He didn't like heights or flying trapeze.

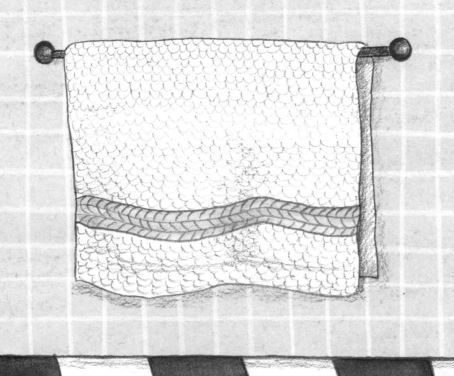

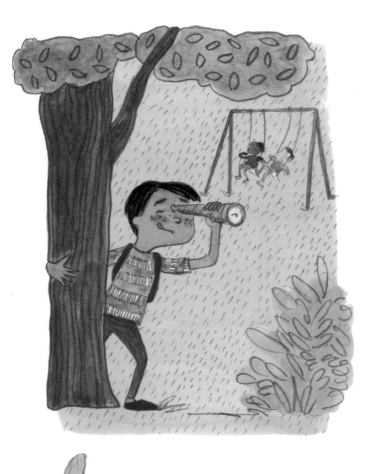
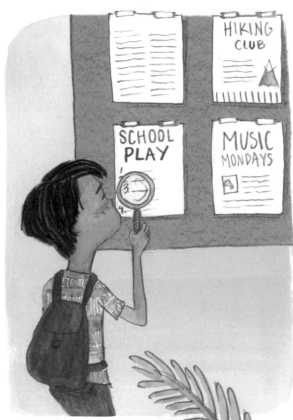

The next day Tyler was on a mission
in search of a special club audition.
He searched the park, the school, the mall. . . .

At the dentist's office, he found a wall.

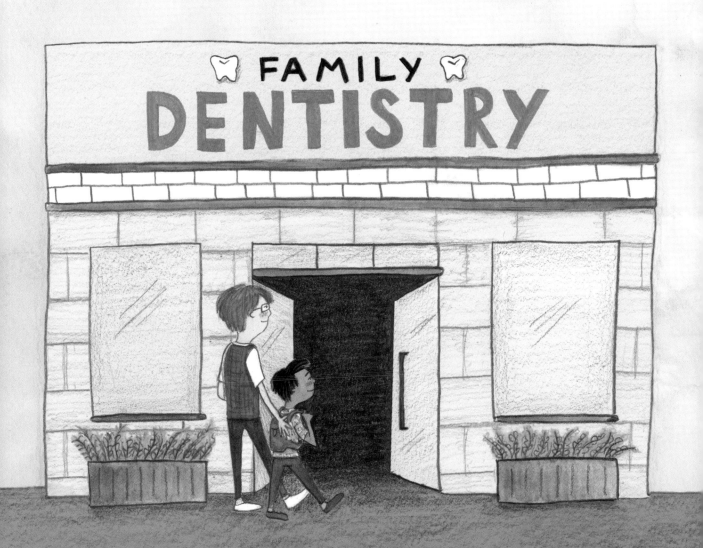

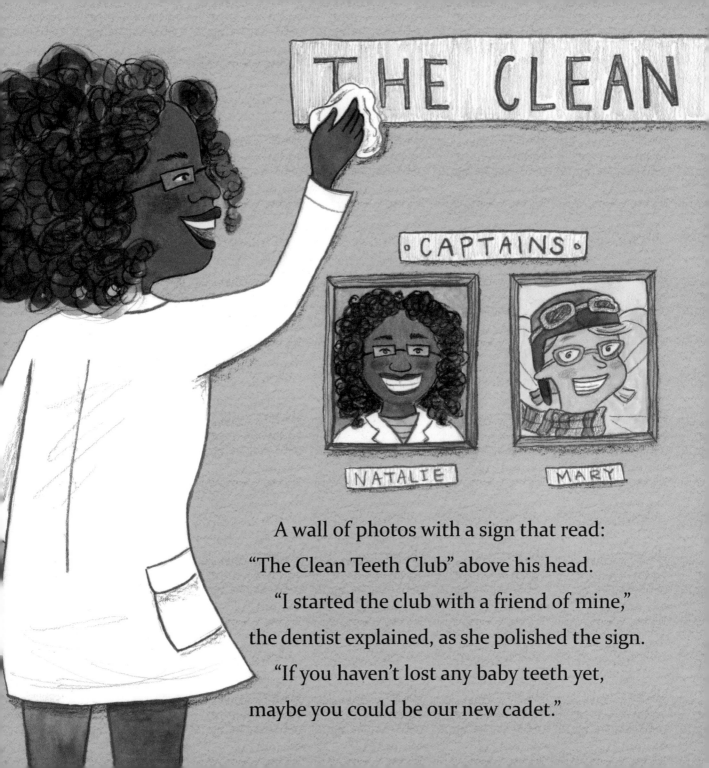

THE CLEAN

•CAPTAINS•

NATALIE

MARY

A wall of photos with a sign that read:
"The Clean Teeth Club" above his head.
   "I started the club with a friend of mine,"
the dentist explained, as she polished the sign.
   "If you haven't lost any baby teeth yet,
maybe you could be our new cadet."

TEETH CLUB

"Just complete three quests before your first loose tooth,
then schedule a cleaning at the reception booth."

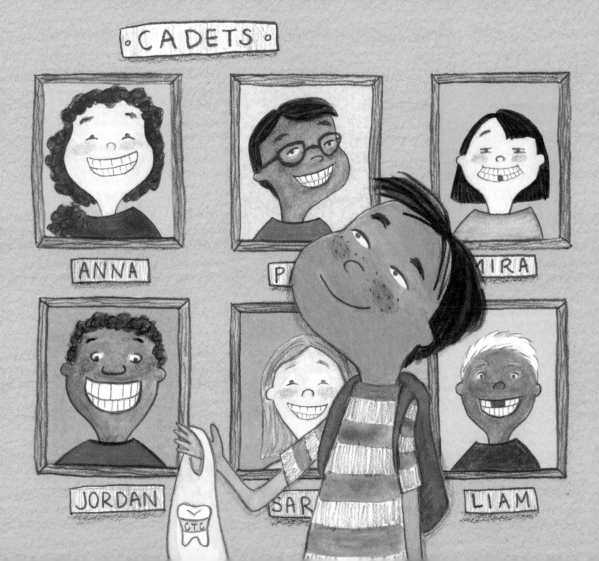

She sent Tyler home with a list of rules,
a brush and a bag of flossing tools.

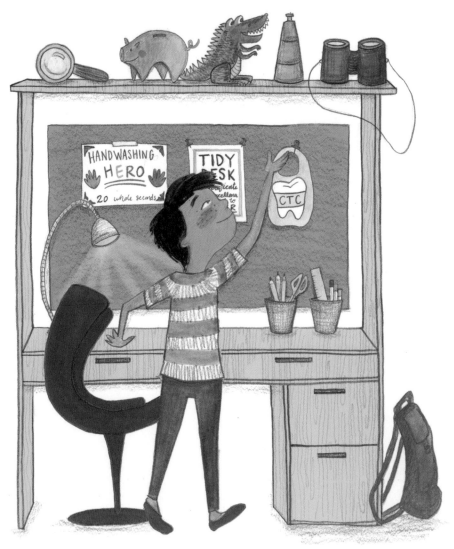

This is it, thought Tyler, *the club for me.*

Three cool quests, and no trapeze!

— The Clean Teeth Club —

QUEST 1:

Brush your teeth twice a day for
two minutes with fluoride toothpaste.

Good Luck! — Captain Mary

Tyler started with quest number one.

Brushing! He thought, *this will be fun. . . .*

. . . but two whole minutes felt really long,
and he must have been doing something wrong,
cause his mouth overflowed with foamy bubbles,
and brushing in circles was giving him troubles.

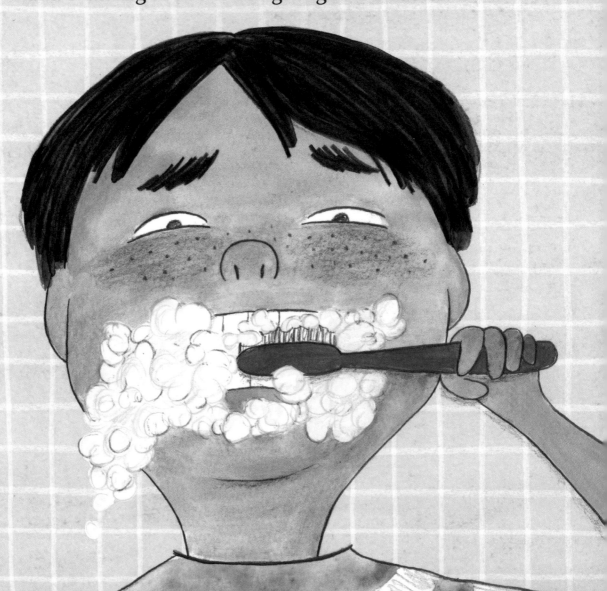

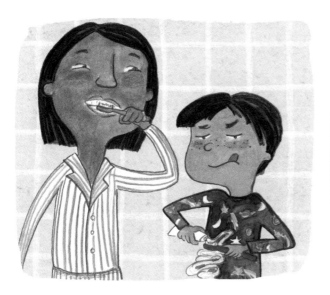
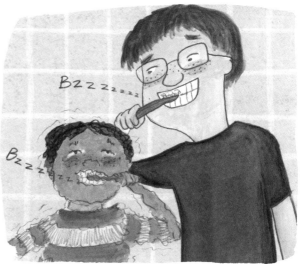

Still, Tyler kept trying, morning and night,
and after three days, he got it right.

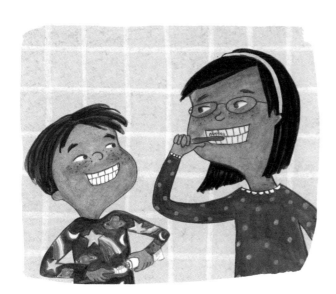
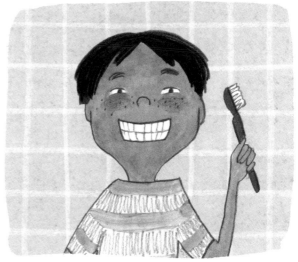

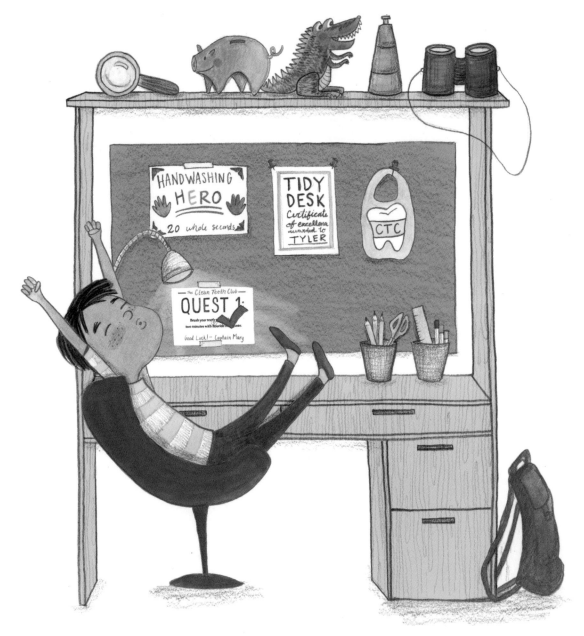

"Quest one done!" Tyler shouted. "Wahoo!"

Then he moved ahead to quest number two.

— The Clean Teeth Club —

QUEST 2:

Floss once a day.

Good Luck! — Captain Mary

Flossing? He thought.

That's easy enough. . . .

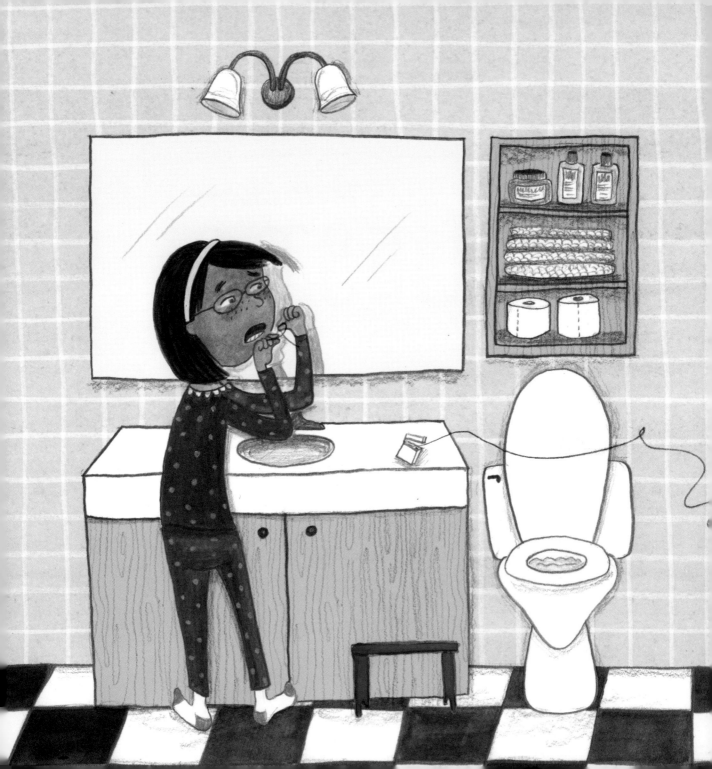

But it turned out flossing was kind of tough.
He followed the steps his dentist had taught,
  but his fingers got tangled in a flossy knot.
He squirmed and jerked to wiggle loose,
  then frowned and said, "Oh, what's the use?"

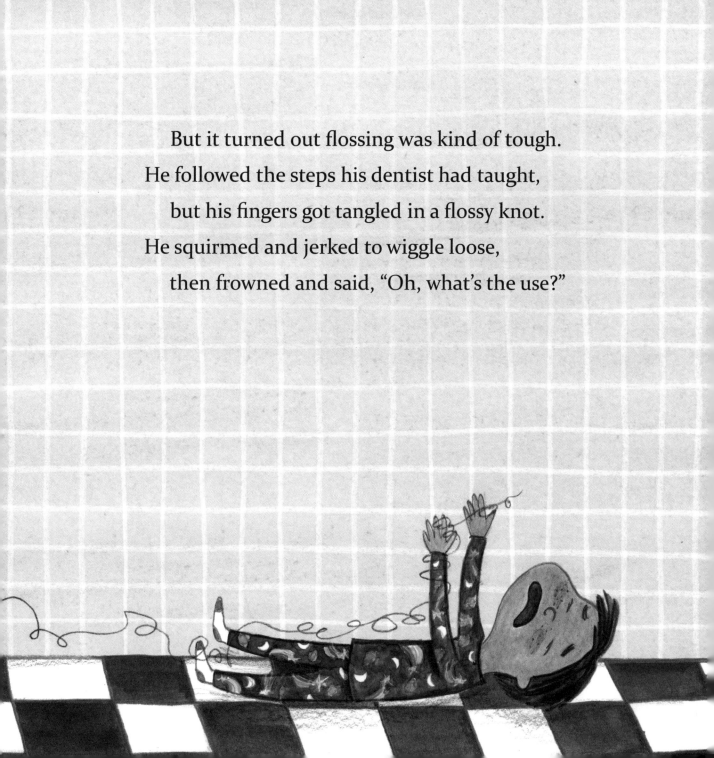

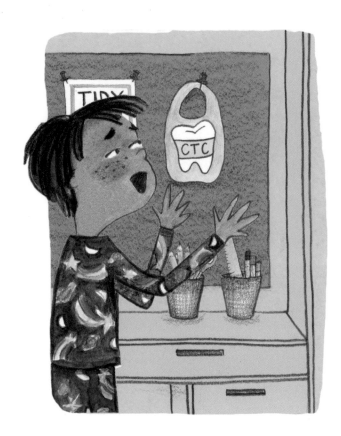

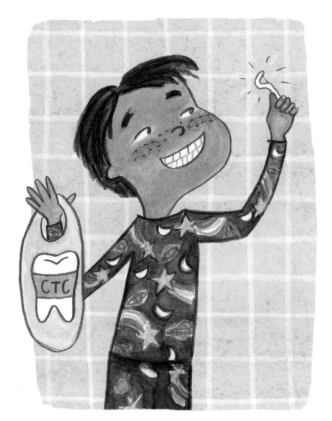

Just as Tyler was about to quit,
he saw the bag and said, "That's it!"
The perfect flossing tools inside
helped Tyler floss his teeth with pride.
Two quests down, only one quest more,
he read the card just as before.

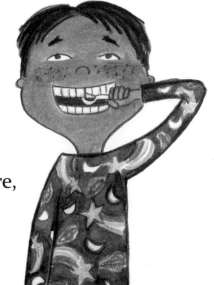

Tyler cried out loud, "Oh noooooo!"

Would all of his favorites have to go?

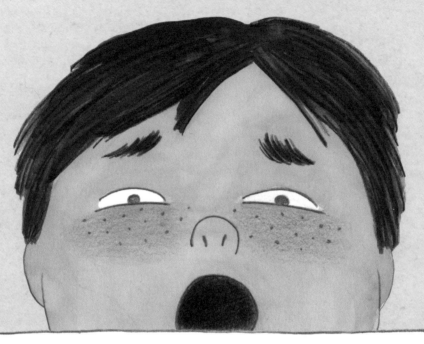

— The Clean Teeth Club —

QUEST 3:

Keep your teeth strong
with healthy snacks.

Good Luck! — Captain Mary

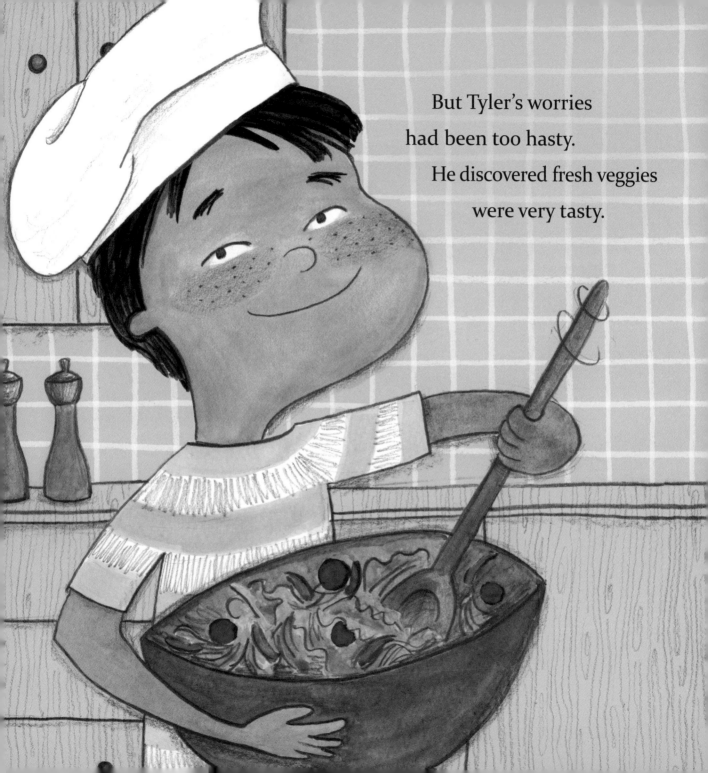

But Tyler's worries
had been too hasty.
He discovered fresh veggies
were very tasty.

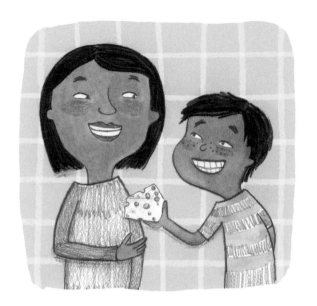
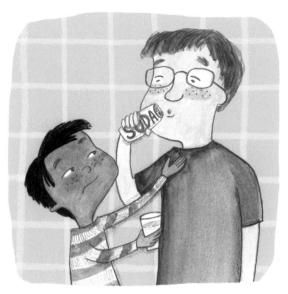

Healthy choices became automatic.

Tyler was soon a health food fanatic.

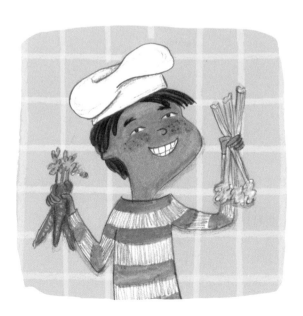
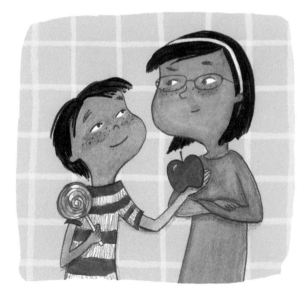

"That's it!" said Tyler. "Quest three is done."

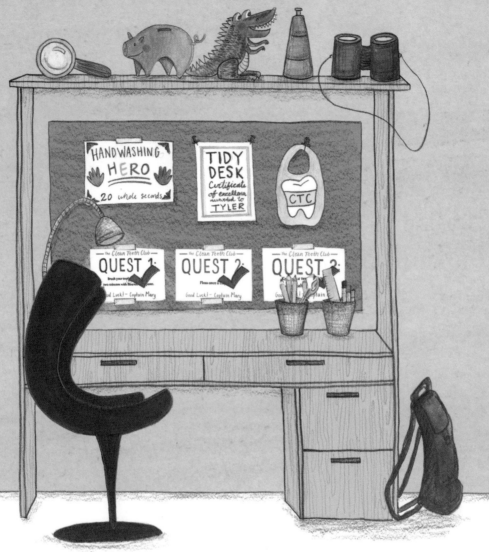

His cleaning was scheduled for Tuesday at one.

He'd pass the inspection, he had no doubt,

then without any warning . . .

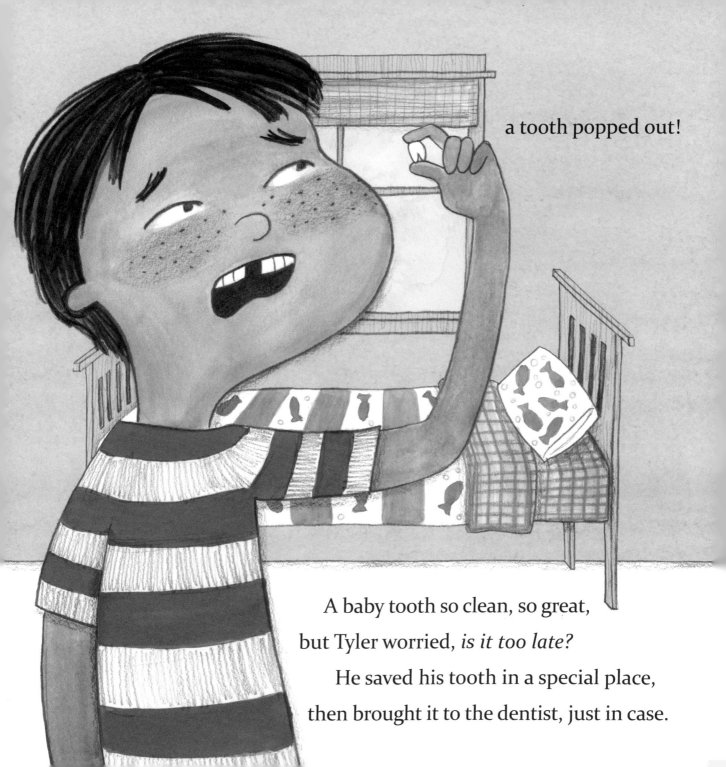

a tooth popped out!

A baby tooth so clean, so great,
but Tyler worried, *is it too late?*
He saved his tooth in a special place,
then brought it to the dentist, just in case.

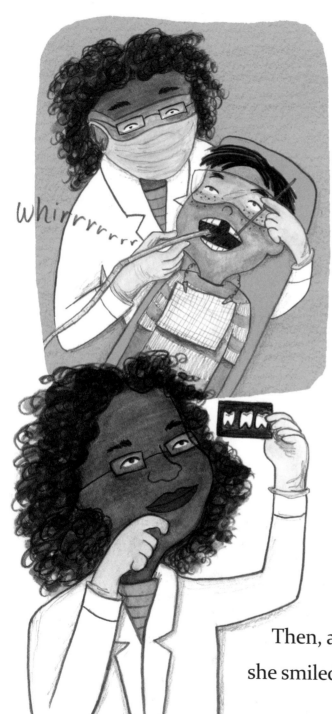

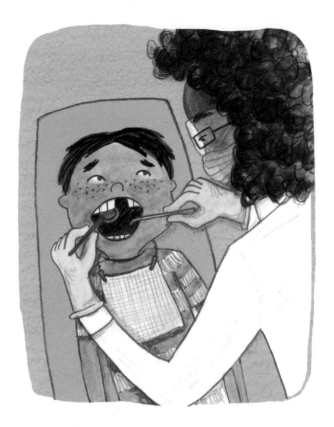

She checked his mouth,
the front, the back.
She took some X-rays,
removed some plaque.

Then, after what felt like one whole year,
she smiled and said, "Don't worry dear."

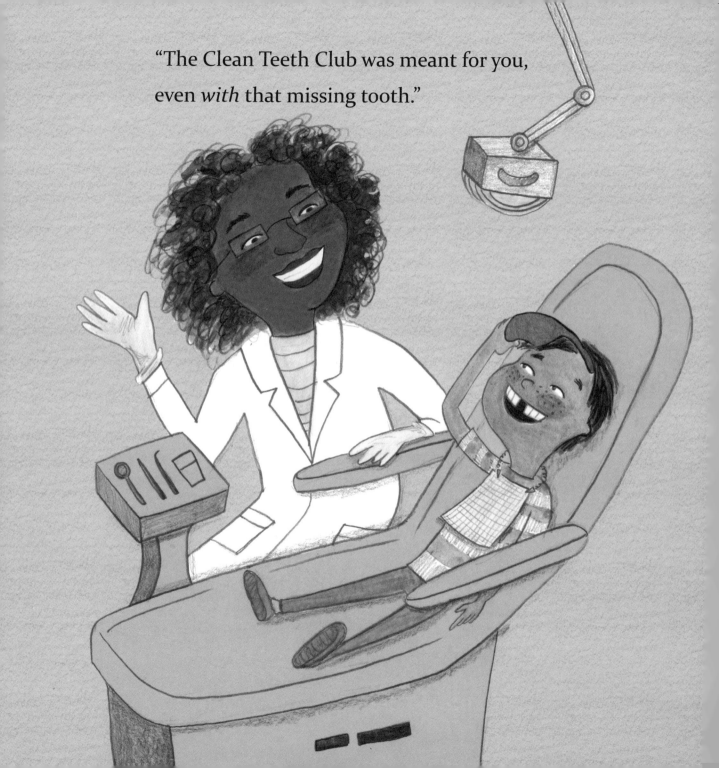

"The Clean Teeth Club was meant for you, even *with* that missing tooth."

THE CLEAN TEETH

· CAPTAINS ·

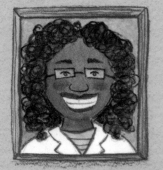

NATALIE

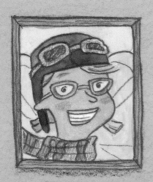

MARY

· CADETS ·

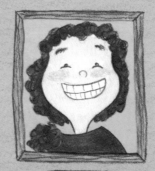

ANNA

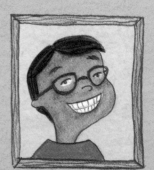

PABLO

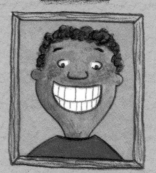

JORDAN

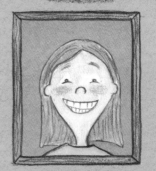

SARAH

And so he made it on the wall,
one big toothless grin and all.

CLUB

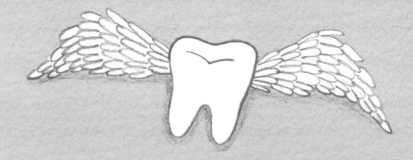

•CREW• •COPILOTS•

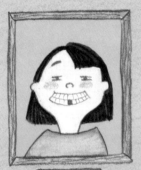
MIRA

TYLER

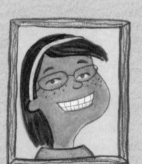

BELLA

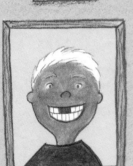
LIAM

MAYA

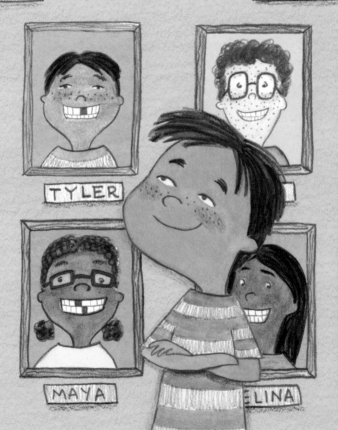

ELINA

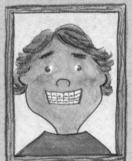
MASON

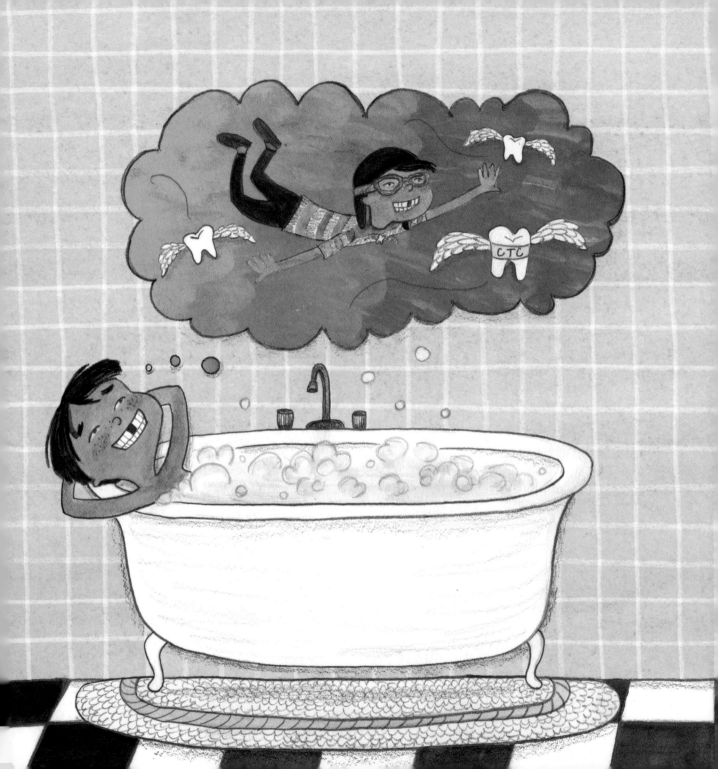

That night while Tyler sat in the tub,

he thought about the Clean Teeth Club.

He wondered about this mysterious Mary . . .

and he said, "I bet she knows the tooth fairy!"

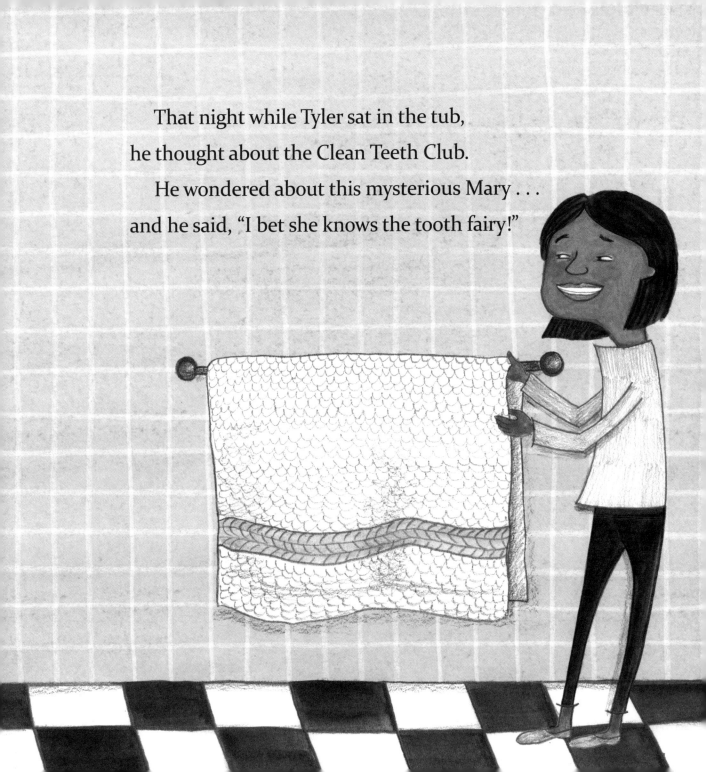

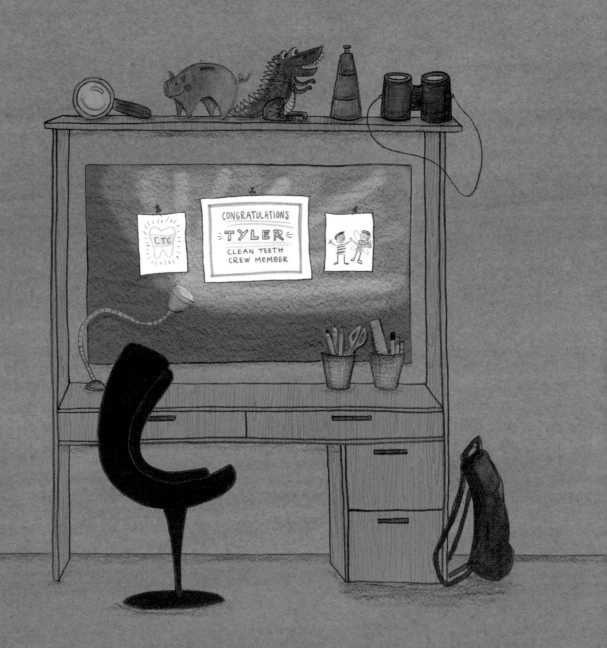

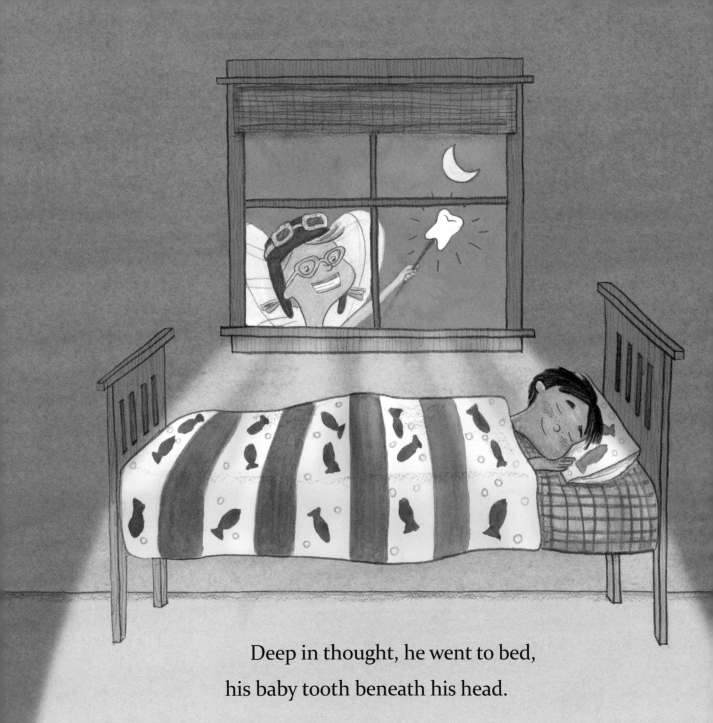

Deep in thought, he went to bed,

his baby tooth beneath his head.

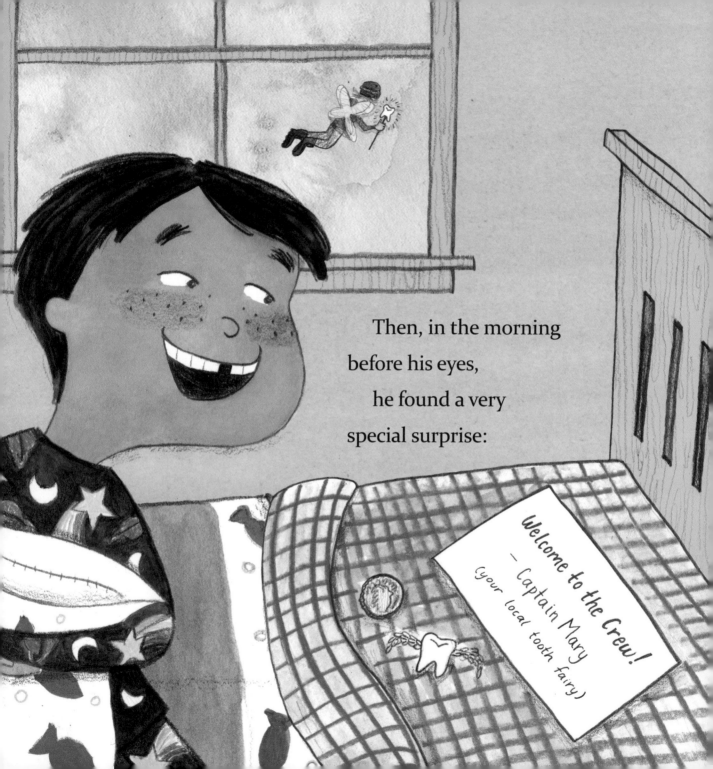

Then, in the morning
before his eyes,
he found a very
special surprise:

Welcome to the Crew!
— Captain Mary
(your local tooth fairy)